GET UP
and
GET MOVING

57
~~56~~ THINGS TO DO

D. A. Featherling

DEDICATION

To all my fellow couch potatoes who also
need to —

Get Up and Get Moving

ACKNOWLEDGMENTS

Thanks to authors Sidney W. Frost, Linda Farmer Harris, and Teresa Lynn for valuable suggestions. Thanks to artist Dave Allred for a fun cover (www.drawnbydave.com). And thanks to Linda Farmer Harris for technical assistance.

Thanks to Joyce Rector for frequently pointing out the benefits of exercise until "I finally got it."

Thanks to Jesus, for creating me 'fearfully and wonderfully made' and for the gift of writing.

INTRODUCTION

As time goes by and our bodies quit obeying our every whim on demand, we discover there are many minutes and hours each day occupied in sitting. Whether it's our favorite recliner, the sofa, or some other comfortable seat, we spend a lot of time without getting up – except to take care of eating and other necessary bodily functions.

I decided it might be of benefit to others who have either accepted, or embraced, the seated quo, for me to take a brief hiatus from my usual authorial pursuits and put out this little volume to provide alternatives to a continuous semi-prone position.

Realizing many of us have health and/or

mobility issues (I have my share), and knowing how much I'd resent some buff, thirty-something telling me to get off my sofa and get moving, I thought it might be more acceptable if one of 'us' offered the information.

I also am aware many are no longer able to do their own housework. Knowing there are things around our homes, be they houses, apartments, or rooms, that others don't normally take care of, I offer this list beyond those types of activities.

I'm sure I've missed some items you may think would be fairly obvious...and if you believe I have, please feel free to email me at dafeatherling@gmail.com and give me your suggestions for additions. If a second book seems warranted, I will feel it's only proper...perhaps even my civic duty...to produce a second volume.

All that said, I realize there are also many who are physically able to find things to do to pass the time, but who may lack the imagination, or the interest in doing so. I hope you, too, will encounter at least a few things in this book to get you up and moving with the best of them.

I am not a medical person, an exercise expert, or any kind of authority on any of this. Simply one person who discovered, after surgery, the more I sat, the less activity I was able to engage in during the months afterward. It took a while for me to figure this out, prodded on by one of my sisters who has a tendency to tell me what I should be doing. She is also, unfortunately, frequently right. I tried exercising daily, which is great, and I still do, but being an author, I have to sit a lot to write books. I needed something more to motivate me to get up off my recliner and do something physical every so often. I can only tell you, it's made a definite difference for the better for me.

If you're concerned you might not be able to perform any of these activities, by all means, don't do them. Check with your doctor first, if you want to. That's always a good idea.

I will refrain from reminding you how unhealthy it is for us to sit so much. Or how much energy and muscle mass we lose by excessive lack of movement. With little activity comes less and less energy and stamina, and therefore, a shorter life span. I'm sure your friendly favorite physician will agree.

If none of the suggestions appeal to you,

perhaps you will find a few hours of enjoyment reading the list, perusing my sometimes snarky comments, or shaking your head anyone would even consider doing these things to get up and get moving.

Enough. Turn the page, dear reader, and enjoy…or employ…the suggestions you find here. You pick…you choose. Or not. Can it get any easier than that? By the way, I'll give you an initial, unnumbered tip. If you find you want to begin using the suggestions without reading the entire book, or even after you've read the book and are ready to begin, you may want to use it as a reference manual as you work.

No problem. Get some wooden clothespins (the kind you mash together), chip bag clips, giant rubber bands, or anything you can use to hold open the pages where you want to read. Be sure to put clips on BOTH sides of the book, because depending how far into the volume you are, the weight of the pages has to be balanced. Clever, hmm?

Now…read on.

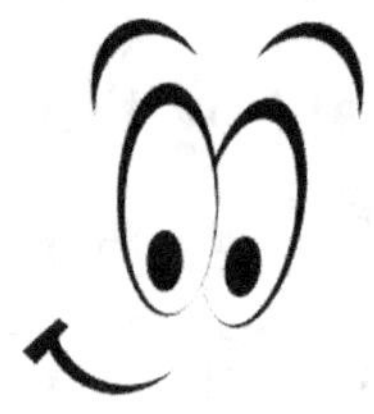

CHAPTER ONE

CLEANING

COMMENTS: You may wonder why I start with one of everyone's least favorite activities. Unless, of course, you are a neat freak, who loves to clean, clean, clean.

If you fall into that category, however, I seriously doubt you'd ever pick up this book, let alone read it. Unless, of course, you've run out of anything to clean and hope to glean a few ideas. If so, welcome, but realize the purpose of these suggestions is not to fuel your unusual behavior.

These are in no particular order, simply listed as they occurred to me. I didn't even try to separate them into similar activities. But I figure you are adults and quite capable of deciding what goes together and what doesn't.

I wouldn't suggest trying to do all these at once. Perhaps one activity in the morning, and if it's a short/easy one, another in the afternoon, if you have no other reason to get up and move around that day.

If you do, pick one and don't be ashamed to let it stretch out over a couple of days or more if needed. We all have our energy levels. Go with yours. I hope, in time, your stamina may increase because you are getting up more frequently. It seems to work that way for me.

1. Plants in the house – Whether silk or real, it's amazing how the little critters collect dust on their leaves/stems. You can buy a fancy spray can of air to remove the dust,

or use a dust cloth, dampened with plain old water and wipe away. You may be surprised how much newer/fresher your plants look after you've done this. Depending on the size/quantity of said plants, you should get in lots of kneeling, stretching, etc. No fair sitting down to do this activity unless you have a legitimate medical reason.

2. Wall switch plates – This is one you can do pretty quickly. It not only keeps your home cleaner, but if you ever decide to put your dwelling on the market, it will add a sparkle buyers will find appealing, Yes, I used to have a home staging business a few years ago, so I know what I'm talking about. Take a Q-tip and your favorite cleaner, or baking soda and water if you're

allergic, and wipe off all the wall switch plates throughout your home. Do the switches, too. It's amazing how fingerprints, smudges, etc. can collect. I'd suggest you do the same for the plates covering electrical outlets, but I'm afraid you'd hurt yourself if you get too close to the plug holes with something wet. Therefore, I do not recommend you worry about it. After all, they're low enough toward the floor few visitors or family will crawl around on their hands and knees to inspect those plates.

3. Frames – Whether you have wall art, pictures, photos, decorative plates, whatever you've hung on your walls, these, too, tend to accumulate a lot of oily dust. Is that an oxymoron or what? It's not

usually visible unless someone gets really close to the item in question or is uncouth enough to run a finger over the surface to see how clean you keep your home. However, a wet cloth with a little soap or your favorite cleaner on it will get rid of the grunge that occurs from hanging on walls. I'd suggest doing one room per day. Of course, you can put as many days in between as you like. If you have multitudes of wall hangings, you may need to take the room in sections, like one wall per session. While taking care of the frames, take a swipe at the art work/pictures themselves. Only takes a few seconds. Just don't rub too hard at oil paintings in case some of the paint should flake off. You wouldn't want to ruin your Rembrandt, would you?

4. Knickknacks – whether you use this term or call them bric-a-brac, we all have our little collectibles on shelves, counters, furniture tops, etc. If you're one of those folks who is actually serious about collecting, and you have myriads of items throughout a room or your entire abode, then I'd suggest professional help.

A-hem. For cleaning, I mean. It would take you entirely too long to do it yourself. For the rest of us, you can again employ a wet cloth (wetted with H_2O or a cleaner) or you can do a thorough job by removing the items and taking them into the kitchen and washing them in soap and water in the sink. Dry before replacing, of course. Don't wash any framing with soap and water, again, of course.

5. Wipe inside shades of floor lamps/table lamps. Critters seem to like weaving webs, dying, etc. inside the shades. **CAUTION:** Do **NOT** touch a hot bulb (even in passing) with a **<u>wet</u>** cloth. It **WILL** explode. I speak from personal experience. Do one room at a time if many lamps, or make lampshade cleaning a single project. Just be sure to turn off the lamps before tackling the chore and give them time to cool. Of course, you could use a dry cloth, but what's the fun in that?

Are you beginning to get inspired? If so, turn to the last page of this volume. There is a checklist available listing all the projects you can see yourself doing. You'll be able to schedule your project when you want. Isn't that great? Just email me and request it.

6. If you have scatter rugs, and most of us do, either vacuum or wash and dry them, depending on manufacturer's

instructions or your own instincts. If you only do one room a day, it shouldn't be too burdensome. You can also take them outside and use the old-fashioned, but still effective, 'shake the goozle out of them' method to rid yourself of dust, dirt, etc. In fact, this is a good way to get a dose of fresh air from time to time as well.

7. Mirror light fixtures – If your balance/coordination is still excellent, get a small footstool or stepladder and clean the light fixtures above your bathroom mirror(s). Turn off the lights and let them cool before cleaning. USE A FLASHLIGHT so you can see to clean and climb. Don't depend on residual light from the bedroom/hallway or whatever is the closest source of illumination for you to be able to see what you're doing. If the flashlight will stand on end, that's a good

way to do it. If not, prop it where it shines in the mirror. The reflected light will help you see. Again, <u>be sure the bulbs are cool before you begin</u>. While you're there, you might clean the top third of the mirror after you get through with the lights. You can do the rest of the mirror from the floor.

8. If you do your own housework, clean the bathroom – sink/counter, toilet space, tub/shower. If energy levels are low, do one fixture per day. Do this weekly. Do it thoroughly. Your bathrooms will sparkle. You might even get nominated for a housekeeping award, if they still give those.

9. Floors – again, if you do your own housework, mop the floors. One per day as you can. Enough said.

10.Same thing for sweeping and/or vacuuming floors. Again, enough said.

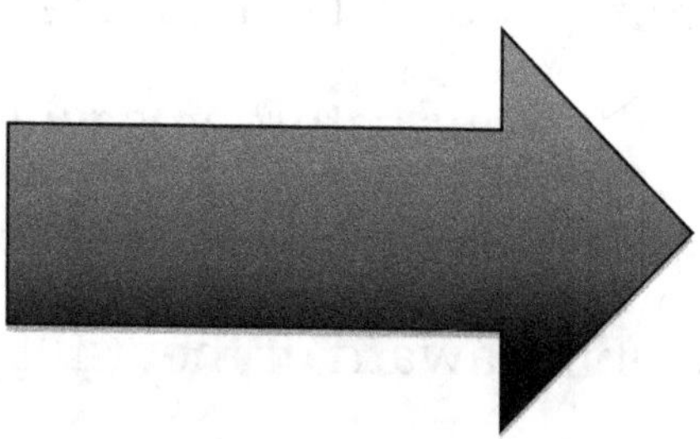

CHAPTER ONE-AND-A-HALF

COMMENT: Hey, it's my book. Besides, you need a page break here to keep you from going to sleep and staying in a seated position even longer. Read on. You're still in the cleaning tips section.

STILL CLEANING

11. If you have shower curtains/liners in your bathtub(s), wipe them clean from time to time, or if you have cloth ones, launder according to instructions. The bottoms of those babies really don't have to stay yellow. You can even put the plastic shower curtains in the washer. Just don't try to dry them in the dryer. You will be

buying a new appliance if you do. Drape the plastic type over the backs of a couple of chairs until they dry, or re-hang them and put the bottom inside the tub and let them drip dry.

12. Clean the TV screen(s), computer/laptop screens, your glasses, camera lenses, tablet or Kindle screens, or your binocular lenses. You don't really use the binoculars from inside your house, do you? Do you? Hmmm. There are all kinds of products available to clean these, up to and including good old-fashioned water on a cloth. It's amazing how clean screens and lenses make a difference in what you see.

13. Stove hood/filter above cook surface – take out the filter. Yes, it will come out, but be careful. If it's been there for a while,

it may have some ragged edges. Soak the filter in soapy water for a bit. Rinse, pat dry and re-insert. While you're letting it soak, wipe the inside of the stove hood, and even the outside with your favorite kitchen cleaner. Mmmm. Looks nice. Beware, though. The filter will be greasy so be sure you get all the grease out before trying to re-insert. The little varmint can be a bit slippery if not thoroughly clean. Just a caution.

Aren't you feeling healthier already? With all the bending, stretching, etc., you're doing, you're exercising places you normally don't use. Good job!

14. Microwave – I discovered this on my own, although I'm sure others already knew, when my cup of water for hot tea insisted on bubbling over in the morning

onto the tray it sat on. Put a full cup of water inside the microwave. Microwave for 2 minutes. <u>Be sure cup handle isn't hot when you remove the cup</u>. There should be water all over the bottom of the appliance, and maybe even some on the sides/top. Unless you have a lot of hardened splatters, a quick wipe with a damp cloth/paper towels should clean things up. It's a quick and easy way to clean the microwave without chemicals. I suspect they'd get in my food…yuck. If you have a removable tray, take it out and clean underneath as well.

15. If you have your own washer/dryer, take a damp cloth and wipe off the tops of the appliances to remove dust buildup. Wait. You aren't through. NOW, open the

lid/door of your washer and dryer one at a time and wipe the rim around where the lid/door shuts. Hmmm. Yes, see all the stuff accumulated in the corners? Of course, while you're there, you might check the filter on the dryer. Unless you clean the filter each time you dry a load of clothes, which I do, you may have lint build up which keeps your appliance from operating at maximum efficiency. Keep a small, stiff vegetable brush nearby to remove the lint in a heartbeat each time you do laundry.

16. Buy a cheap, microfiber duster (dollar stores are your friend) and use to run over the blinds in each room. Do one room a day. Or a week. Turn the slats in one direction, swipe the duster over them.

Reverse the slats, do the other side. Give a little swipe at the windowsill while you're there. Where DO these critters come from and why select MY windowsills as the place to die? Now, don't you feel good about yourself?

17. Use the same duster, or your vacuum attachment, to clean your air conditioning duct vents. If you have to climb on something to reach ones in the ceiling, you may want to have someone else (i.e., younger/steadier) do it for you, but if there are floor-level ones, you can do those. Be prepared, though. Much of the dust is a bit oily and tends to cling to the vents. It may take a bit more vigor than you'd expect to get rid of it. A bit of cleaner on your cloth will help remove it.

Or use a vegetable-brush. Scrub away.

18. Use the long, skinny attachment (crevice cleaner) that fits on your vacuum. Fire up said vacuum and use it to clean the crevices of sofa and chairs. You'd be surprised how many crumbs can collect in those areas. You don't eat in your living room? Really? Huh. I thought everybody did. You may also discover things smaller than a breadbox, which have been lost for several weeks or months. At the least, there may be some pocket change there to reward you.

19. Exercise equipment – Exercise bikes, Total Gyms, treadmills, etc. They all need to be cleaned from time to time. Use a damp cloth or favorite cleaner to clean any display screen on the equipment. You can

also use sanitizing wipes to clean handles, seats, pedals, etc. These items get dusty, too. Unless, of course, they have become handy storage for discarded clothes, etc. In that case, donate them to your local thrift store. The exercise equipment...not the clothes. Well, maybe the clothes, too.

You should be figuring out that simply standing up is insufficient. You also need to walk, bend, flex, stretch, etc. Move in any direction you can do safely and watch how you loosen up those out-of-use muscles.

If you've ever watched professional house cleaners, you can pick up some pretty clever tricks. They never spray furniture polish on a surface to clean. Instead, they spray the dust cloth they are using and wipe. Uses a whole lot less polish, goes a lot faster, and keeps more chemical odor from being put into the air. Neat!

CHAPTER TWO

EDIT

COMMENTS: Since many of us dread the words "get rid of", I've chosen to use the term "edit" rather than "delete" to accomplish the same purpose. I mean the same thing.

Of course, you may not need to sacrifice your stuff…but you do need to review it, decide what's really necessary and what's not.

Looking is the only way to tell and it may give you a trip down memory lane, remind you of something you forgot to do, find an item you've wondered about…all sorts of good can come from "editing". It's also an opportunity to contribute to charitable organizations that accept donations of gently-used items, or you'll be amazed at how many trash bags you may fill to put out for the weekly garbage collection if the items aren't up to donation.

Let's face it. We all have more stuff than we need, use, or even want. Why not let the decision to get up and get moving afford you the opportunity to organize your life a bit? At worst, "editing" will give you more room to buy more stuff. There. Does that make it feel better?

1. Review your collections of DVDs, videos, and CDs. Weed out the ones you never listen to. Yes, they might be worth something to a collector, but who do you know who fits that category? Not all discards are really someone else's treasure. If you absolutely love eBay and putting

things on it, by all means go ahead and offer your Roy Rogers collection of early TV shows. I bought one for my grandson. He's never watched it. I watched one episode and wondered why I thought it was so wonderful back in the day. The box lived on my DVD tower until I finally edited it. Then Roy and several others went to the thrift store. Bound to be a kid out there somewhere who still likes old Westerns. *SPECIAL HINT*: You can also do this on the DVR on your TV. It only holds so many episodes and you may need to clear some out to make room for more. A word to the wise from one whose recording space sat at 92% full until a few days ago.

2. Clean out closets — I never said you'd

LOVE all these suggestions, now did I? Do this one closet at a time. If you're like most of us, your wardrobe has meandered into more than one closet in more than one room. Here's the key: Get rid of anything you haven't worn in TWO YEARS. Wait for six months…then do it again. Eliminate anything one-year-old with the tags still on it. It's okay as long as you don't possess more than four tagged items. We all occasionally make shopping mistakes. If you have more than four still-tagged items, take someone you trust with you whenever you shop.

3. Go through your shoes (boots, sandals, etc.) Do you really need two pairs of swim shoes? Won't one do? Go through the footwear, edit as many as possible using

the 1-2 year rule mentioned above. While you're editing, check and see if any of your footwear needs cleaning or repairing. If so, clean or take for repair. If an item isn't in good condition, consider discarding. I know they're comfy, but will you really EVER wear them again?

4. Go through your belts/scarves/neckties – Edit as many as possible, again using the 1-2 year rule.

5. Go through your wardrobe/armoire – Hah! You thought I'd forgotten it, didn't you? Counts the same as closets. Edit via the 1-2 year rule.

If you've put any of the suggestions made thus far into practice on any sort of regular basis, you should be able to tell some difference in how you feel. How you can move more easily. Do you?

6. In the kitchen, pull out ALL your plastic

storage containers…yes, **all** of them. Take out all the lids you have for such containers. Now…match them! Hmm! Is there a game show possibility here? If they take up the entire counter surface in the kitchen and spill over into another room, consider having a party and let the 'match 'em' game be the entertainment. Just a thought. Discard the extra lids and the containers for which there are no lids (where DO those things go?). Either donate them or recycle them…your call.

7. Knickknacks/bric-a-brac — Yep. You cleaned them earlier. But have you ever tried rearranging them? Put things on different shelves, in different rooms. It's amazing what changing things around does to give a room a fresh new look

without spending a penny.

8. Jewelry — Ladies, sort through your costume jewelry and take the unwanted items to a thrift store. Or donate them to a nursing home for game prizes or to a church for prizes for events. Are you really going to wear the item again? Especially since it's been out of style for two or three years? Okay. Ten or fifteen years.

9. Men — do the same thing with items on your valet. Yes, it's okay to go beyond jewelry. Whatever you stow on top of the valet is fair game for editing.

10. Magazines — sort through the magazines on your coffee table, end tables, yes, dare I say it, in your bathroom? Decide which ones you really will read. Recycle or donate the rest to libraries or nursing homes. Some

teachers of lower grades would like to have them for class projects as well.

11. Edit bath towels, hand towels, wash cloths, dish towels, dish cloths, bathroom rugs/toilet seat/tank covers. Discard ones that are frayed, worn thin, torn, etc. You can use some of them as cleaning rags for other projects or simply discard. Only throwing away the first one hurts.

> If your shoes tend to get stinky, just sprinkle some baking soda inside and leave it until you're ready to wear them again. Tap out the leftover soda and wear.

CHAPTER THREE

EDIT/ORGANIZE

COMMENTS: Just when you thought I was going to run out of ideas. Tch. Tch. Ye of little faith. Sometimes editing isn't enough. You also need to organize after you edit. Granted this is a more serious project than editing and discarding, but I know you can handle it.

If you need to, make it a two-part project. I realize we may all be operating with limited energy. I'm just trying to give you reasons to get up and move around occasionally, not exhaust you.

The following ideas will definitely bring some order to your home and enhance your health at the same time. Onward....

1. Dresser drawers — ugh. You're already dreading this one, aren't you? That's okay. Do them one at a time. That's right. You don't have to do the whole piece of furniture at the same time. If you really feel enthused and energetic, do two drawers. Edit the stuff you never use. Be ruthless. Organize whatever's left into neatness. And remember, you can switch stuff around and put it in different drawers for convenience or for a change of pace. Just be sure the first few times you try to find something you have a light on so you don't pick up the wrong item.

2. Chest of drawers — next most-dreaded project. (And by the way, it isn't 'chester drawers'). Do the same as in number 1. Be sure you can still wear items stored there.

Do the same for any armoire or wardrobe as well. I suspect there are all kinds of clothing and other items you don't need/use.

3. Bedside tables — As long as you're on a roll, edit and organize there as well. You may be amazed what you'll find. Or thought you'd lost.

4. Medications — Go through all your prescription/non-prescription meds in bathrooms, bedside tables, kitchen, one day at a time, if needed. Get rid of out-of-date items. Check with your pharmacist if you aren't sure. Organize the others to be able to easily find them.

Whether up and down, or back and forth, various movements are building you some stamina. Being on our feet more helps, too. Are you telling a difference for the better? Keep it up.

5. Jewelry — Ladies, you may want to do this one first before you tackle number 8 under "Edit." Go through all your jewelry, costume or real, and match jewelry to the remaining clothes you now have in your closets.

    Discard jewelry that no longer goes with anything, or items you're tired of, or plan to leave someone in your will. Either go ahead and give it to them now and enjoy watching them wear it, or if worth more than sentimental value, put it in a safety deposit box in your financial institution.

    Keep only those items that actually go with something you have to wear or make a list of the jewelry you're keeping and take it with you the next time you go clothes shopping. Try to match what you have with what you need to buy. If you can't find an outfit to match, you probably don't need to keep the jewelry.

Organize your keepers into matching pairs/sets while you're at it. Put necklaces, bracelets, brooches, earrings that go together in the same place in the jewelry box. It's amazing how easy it'll be to spot what you want rather than having to rummage through everything to find the rest of a set. If you have to invest in another jewelry box, feel free to do so. After all, more sometimes gets you better organized.

6. Books — Sort through the books in your bookcases. Edit for ones you know you will read or re-read. I have a number of favorites I actually do re-read from time to time, so I keep those in case they become hard/impossible to find in the future. Most

have. Donate your discards to the public library, church library, or a nursing home Nursing homes love to have books for their residents to read.

7. Under the kitchen sink — can you believe all the stuff down there? Edit and organize what's left. You might check those expiration dates, too.

8. Coat closet — ah, forgot about that one, didn't you? Edit your hanging garments as well as what's on the shelf/shelves. Organize/rearrange/discard/donate.

9. Spices in kitchen — I know, everybody tells you to do this one, but have you ever tried it? Amazing how much shelf space you'll free up. You'll also be surprised how much of this stuff has expired because you only needed a particular spice for one

recipe…that you haven't made again in the last three years. Edit and organize. Check expiration dates. Note to self whether or not to buy again depending on how much you enjoyed the original dish.

10. Items in pantry — What can I say? Edit, organize, check expiration dates. If you do have unexpired items, but know you won't likely ever eat them, consider donating to your local food pantry.

Evidently, rubber gloves attract pet hair like a magnet. Rub your gloved hands over the surface to be cleaned and watch the pet hair cling. When you've removed as much as you can, go to a sink full of water and wash your gloved hands. Most of the pet hair will float to the top.

CHAPTER FOUR

CLEAN/EDIT

COMMENTS: There she goes again! (you're thinking). Now she wants to clean *and* edit! No, I'm not a fanatic, I'm just trying to give you some ideas…and maybe a bit of incentive…to get up and get moving.

I can tell you from personal experience it isn't a whole lot of fun to develop other ailments because you sat too much and caused them to occur. Cut me some slack and read on for more ideas for projects.

1. One cabinet at a time, one bathroom at a time, remove everything from bathroom shelves (whether in a cabinet or out of

one). Edit and replace the rest. Wipe shelves and the bottom of the cabinet with a damp cloth before replacing items. Check expiration dates if there is one, particularly items in the cabinet(s) under the sink. Even bath stuff can get old, and, if it's scented, lose or change its fragrance.

By the way, I'm aware that some days, you may not feel like doing anything but sitting. It happens to me, too. Use your brain or fingers, instead. Anything to keep your mind occupied and moving when your body needs a break.

Getting tired of having packages of meat scattered throughout my freezer, I went to the dollar store (love those places) and bought a plastic shoebox storage box. I put it on one side of the freezer and stowed all the individual packages. If you have a lot of packages or a lot of room in your freezer, use two storage boxes. Simple!

CHAPTER FIVE

GENERAL

COMMENTS: you're probably wondering why I stick this in the middle of a list instead of waiting until the end. Good question. On the other hand, why not? The topic seems to fit, if not the category. Stiffen that upper lip, put away your critique cap, and continue reading.

1. If you have several items to carry from one room to another (stuff to put away, or new purchases you need to stow [tch, tch, *more to edit?*]), make separate trips with each one. Keeps you on your feet, therefore off your chair, longer. And, you won't harm

your neck, back or shoulders by carrying too heavy a load.

If your pet wets on your carpet/rug, try sprinkling baking soda over the wetted area. Let dry and vacuum. Most/all of smell should be gone. Your visitors will appreciate it.

CHAPTER SIX

KINDNESS

COMMENTS: I could probably add many more suggestions to the kindness list, but the idea behind this volume is to get you moving around to be more mobile. If you have other ways of showing kindness to others, good for you. If not, this may get you thinking in that direction. It doesn't matter if it's random or deliberate, kindness is still kindness. Fact.

1. Go to a dollar store (it gets you up and out) and buy $1 - $10 (or whatever you can afford) worth of useful gadgets, containers, etc. Put a small ribbon on each one and leave outside the front door of neighbors,

anonymously. This works especially well if you live in an apartment/retirement center. Hang on the doorknob if the doors have them. Be sure to put a ribbon on them to indicate it's a gift. Otherwise the recipient may think someone lost it and turn it in or trash it. The possibilities for these little gifts are endless. As are the dollar stores.

2. Do the same thing, only use greeting cards ("Thinking of You," "Hello," all kinds of categories abound). Either use the ones you've accumulated over the years and never have sent/given, or back to the dollar store where you can buy most cards for fifty cents each. Sometimes they even have boxes of cards for a dollar. If you're really talented, create your own cards.

That's even more special.

To clean your garbage disposal occasionally, dump a tray or two of ice cubes in the sink, shove them inside the disposal (while it's off, of course), then turn on the water gently, and run the disposal until the ice is ground up. To freshen, whenever I peel an orange, lemon, or lime, I take the peelings and run them through the disposal. Gives a nicer odor for a while than old food. You may want to take half the orange peel, put it in a plastic bag and store in the fridge for a week or so, then you'll have peeling to use to freshen even if you don't have/eat a citrus fruit that day.

CHAPTER SEVEN

FOOD

COMMENTS: Everyone's eating habits are different. Depending upon what yours are, the following suggestions may, or may not, apply. However, I hope you are eating at least a few fruits and veggies each week…better yet, according to the experts, each day.

I personally like them and have found ways to preserve them for maximum freshness. I like them, but I don't particularly like prepping them frequently, so I've tried to discover ways to extend time between that cleaning chore as much as possible. Hope these will work for you.

1. Buy (and eat) lots of veggies that need to be cleaned before being consumed – lettuce, celery, radishes, carrots, etc. Wash and store them in plastic bags lined in the bottom with three layers of paper towels. Paper towels should extend up the sides about four inches on each side besides lining the bottom. Put another three layers of towels over the top of the cleaned veggies and tuck in the edges so no produce is seen. Squeeze out the excess air as you zip closed. Store bag(s) in the fridge for up to three weeks. Yep, they'll really keep that long. Works especially well for lettuce.

2. Do not buy pre-cut fruit – as attractive as it appears. Instead, buy the stuff you have to prep to eat. Pre-wash strawberries,

blackberries, blueberries, etc. and line a plastic container with two or three thicknesses of paper towels. No, I don't own stock in a paper towel company, I just find the things extremely useful. Put the washed fruit, after blotting it as dry as possible without squishing it, inside on the towels. Put another two or three thicknesses of paper towels on top. Fold as needed to fit container. Put the lid on the container and flip it upside down and store in fridge. This also works well with melons of all kinds. Change the paper towels on top (after container is flipped right side up) when they get moist and replace with new, dry thicknesses. You shouldn't have to replace the bottom layer, it usually lasts throughout the time it takes to eat the contents of the container. Melons will have to be done more frequently at first since they're juicier. Fruit stored this way has lasted me for two or three weeks. Honest!

Standing up to do all this prepping is getting you moving around. Keep up the good work.

3. Check your refrigerator at least every two to three weeks (Okay. Once a month, if you insist) for containers/packages with mold in them (unless you really *are* conducting a scientific experiment requiring mold). Once a month, check your condiments, jams/jellies, milk, etc. for expiration dates. It's amazing how many times we buy things, but don't eat as fast as we thought we would. Do NOT eat expired products unless you really like and miss seeing your local EMS responders.

> If you've scorched food in a pot or pan and usual methods of loosening up the overcooked food isn't getting you anywhere, try ketchup. Because tomatoes are so highly acidic, in many cases the food is eaten away and you can wash and rinse as usual. No guarantee, of course.

How Long Should I Keep It?

FOOD	SHELF LIFE AFTER OPENING
Ketchup	4-6 months in refrigerator
Jelly	1 year in refrigerator
Mustard	6-8 months refrigerated
Broth	2 days in refrigerator
Peanut Butter	2-3 months
Mayonnaise	2 months in refrigerator
All-purpose Flour	10-15 months
Brown Rice	6 months in refrigerator
Vegetable Oil	3 months in pantry, 6 months in refrigerator
Olive Oil	12-18 months
Vinegar	6 months

CHAPTER EIGHT

OUTDOORS

COMMENTS: If you are fortunate enough to be able to do yard work, or have outdoor plants, good for you. You probably aren't spending much time in your chair as a result.

However, if you really don't/can't do outside stuff on a regular basis, some of the following suggestions may get you outdoors occasionally to enjoy the beauties of nature.

Don't hurt yourself. If you have yard people who do the big jobs, and only have a few outdoor plants you care for, that works. Some of us furnish a smorgasbord for mosquitoes every time we go outside with any piece of skin showing...and we live in an area where mosquitoes also live, almost year around.

For those of us with this situation, buy a couple of silk flower bushes (back to the dollar store), take off the tags, suit up in your outdoor protection gear, and run outside and stick them in a planter filled with dirt.

Change the flowers or greenery with the seasons (you only have to do this about four times a year. Unless you're really obsessed with holidays, then you may want to make it six or eight times).

1. If able, trim bushes, weed flower beds, prune trees, rake and bag leaves. You obviously don't need to be reading this book if you can do all of it, but if you get bored easily, especially when indoors, you may still find something of value to do.

2. Clean the light fixtures on your front porch, outside your garage doors, on the back deck/patio/door. Remember the hot light bulb warning from before. A spray with cleaner or the old soap and water thing work equally well. Don't be too surprised at the amount of grime you find. After all, it IS outdoors.

3. Check your welcome/outdoor mats. Clean, or if hopeless, replace.

4. Window screens — Take a brush or wet cloth and clean the bottom half. After all, how many people are tall enough to look through the top half of your windows? Don't, however, go climbing around on things to do this and get hurt.

5. Pull dead blossoms/leaves off plants (if on patio or deck); otherwise let them fall off.

Nature has its own methods of handling them.

6. If you have a bird feeder(s), clean them every three weeks. It's recommended by most manufacturers…and the budgies appreciate it. Wouldn't you?

7. If you have a bird bath…DEFINITELY clean it every few days, if not daily. Many critters will use it or wash stuff in it. After all, the expression "dirty bird" originated for a reason. And they weren't just talking about personal bird hygiene. Have you ever watched a blackbird/crow/raven try to rinse dog food pellets in a bird bath? Yuck.

8. If you have patio/deck furniture, clean it occasionally, especially after bad weather or before a change of season. Watch for

mold on cushions. If that happens, you may need to replace them.

9. Sweep deck/patio/by back door weekly or every couple of weeks. Get rid of leaves, twigs, dead critters, etc. Bug-type, of course. Any bigger critters, call local animal control.

10. Mulch – mulch is your friend. It can cover a multitude of issues – spread it in flower beds to help control weeds/trees/etc. from coming up. It also adds a nice touch to the outside of your home. If you're using it strictly for a decorative touch, a THIN layer is sufficient. If you're doing it for weed control, thicker is better.

If you participate in even half or a fourth of these suggestions, I suspect you'll see improvement in how you feel. Am I right? Of course I'm right.

To prevent getting dirt under your fingernails while you work in the garden, draw your fingernails across a bar of soap. You'll actually seal the undersides of your nails so dirt won't be able to collect beneath them. When you've finished those garden chores, use a nailbrush to remove the soap and your nails will be nice and clean. Clever, huh?

AND NOW...THE END...

Hopefully, you've hung in here with me to reach this point. Yes, I realize I didn't cover everything that could be done. But...there's possibly going to be book two...remember? Your comments, suggestions, or tips are welcome. Email them to me. In the meantime, get up off your...seating and do get moving. You and your body will be glad you did.

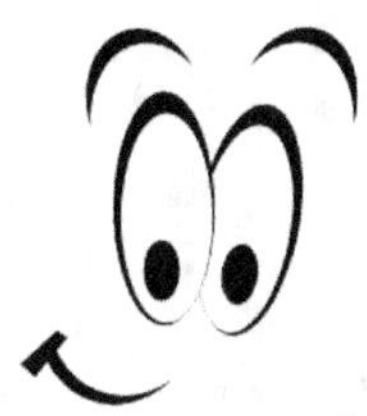

NOW TRULY...THE END

In case you get bored
while you <u>are</u> sitting down,
let me offer you some diversion.

Following is a list of my
Fiction/Non-Fiction books,
and
a few free chapters as a sample
of some of the different genres
in which I write.

After all, we might as well
enjoy our 'down' time.
Right?

BOOKS BY
D. A. FEATHERLING

Mystery

IT'S MURDER AT THE OFFICE SERIES
It Adds Up to Murder (Book 1)
Bubble, Bubble, Toil and…Murder! (Book 2)

STAGED FOR MURDER SERIES
Murder Outside the Box (Book 1)
Conventional Murder (Book 2)

Romantic Comedy/Romance

Sauce for the Goose
Kissing Frogs
Double Trouble
Making Over Caro
Friendly, Michael

End Times Fiction

OUT OF TIME SERIES
Time Out (Book 1)
Double Time (Book 2)
End of Time (Book 3)

YA/Adult Fiction

TIME GAME SERIES
Eye of the Storm: The First Token (Book 1)
Mission to Mars: The Second Token (Book 2)
The Lost City of Acara: The Third Token (Book 3)
My Spy: The Fourth Token (Book 4)
Chisholm Trail Showdown: The Fifth Token (Book 5)

Non-Fiction

Who Killed Ben Miller & Death of a Juror
Write On! Giving 7th & 8th Grade School Presentations
Writing a Book - Giving 9th–12th Grade School Presentations

BIOGRAPHY

D. A. (Dorothy) Featherling writes in multiple genres. She has published adult mysteries, romantic comedies, end times fiction and a romance.

Her non-fiction books include a 1930s cold case murder, and two e-books on giving grade school presentations.

Most recently, she is writing a time travel adventure series (SciFi/Time Travel for ages 9-99). A thirteen-book series is planned. A game (*Time Game)* is already published and available on her websites.

Her administrative years in corporations, state agencies, and a university physics research center, and as owner of a home staging business, have given her a multitude of ideas and characters for her novels.

Her nasty habit of aging has provided her with plenty of incentive and reasons for producing this volume.

She has also written numerous technical pieces and has won awards for fiction, journalism, and public speaking. D.A. now lives in Georgetown, Texas and appears and/or speaks at events for clubs, civic organizations, churches, and schools upon request.

WEBSITES: www.dafeatherling.com
www.timegameseries.com

E-MAIL: dafeatherling@gmail.com

MYSTERY

SPECIAL EXCERPT

Abigail Newhouse hopes her life remains peaceful now she's managing a local antique mall. When murder occurs, however, she still wants to help solve the case. Homicide Lieutenant Nick Vaughn doesn't want Abby involved. Will her pursuit of the truth sidetrack their relationship? And will she be able to escape with her life if she faces the killer in a deadly showdown?

Read on for a portion of Chapter One

Bubble, Bubble, Toil and...Murder

(Book 2, "It's Murder at the Office" Series)

by D.A. Featherling

CHAPTER 1

"Make sure I get it or you may not celebrate another birthday."

The balding man's reddened face, bulging eyes, and line of spittle dribbling down his chin made the threat believable.

My thumping heart and dry mouth didn't make it easy to respond in a soothing tone. "I've told you before, Mr. Simms. I don't have the authority to do that."

"You get it, then, Missie, or you're gonna answer to *me*." His stabbing forefinger added emphasis. "You talk to your boss and tell her if I don't get my way there'll be more trouble than she ever dreamed."

Another glare, more drool before he wheeled and marched his skinny five feet seven inches toward the front door.

Had I come as close to disaster as it sounded? Was Ronald Simms really dangerous or only spouting off?

I couldn't make promises to him. I'm simply a temp filling in as assistant manager in *The Oaken Bucket* antique mall.

I drew a deep breath, then another.

My pulse slowed to something approaching normal as I headed toward the front of the shop. It was past time for a break.

I refused to believe Simms might actually carry out his threats simply because he wanted preference on renting an extra booth in the mall. At least, I hoped not. I wasn't being paid enough to deal with half-crazed vendors like him. Of course, I knew if I walked out of the job early it would leave Elise Lindsey in one huge predicament, but my demise wouldn't exactly make my life more appealing, either.

Mercy. The trials and tribulations of Abigail Newhouse, temporary worker. I'd already discovered there could be few dull moments working in such positions. Now it sounded like my life might be in jeopardy. Again.

I called to Gerianne, the brunette part-time student who helped out after school and on Saturdays. "I'm going for a cup of coffee. I'll be back in ten or fifteen minutes."

She looked up from the homework she had spread on the counter and waved.

I fast-paced toward the coffee shop a few doors away. At this point, only a double mocha raspberry latte would soothe my jangled nerves. And maybe a quick chat with my favorite police lieutenant.

The latte produced the desired results. Unfortunately, Detective Nick Vaughn was out of the office. I sighed. Talking with Nick always made me stronger, more in control of things.

Ever since he'd rescued me from being shot during my last long-term temp job, the casual relationship we'd had until then had become a little more serious.

I still didn't know where our relationship would go…or where we both wanted it to go. I did know I enjoyed his company more than any man's in a long time. His understanding and attention had gone a long way in helping me get over the lingering effects of losing a good university job with outstanding benefits.

Since I'd been unable to find anything comparable on or off campus, I'd taken a job as a temporary worker and discovered I could not only make a decent living, but that I enjoyed the challenge of adapting to new environments and people and making a difference for the better.

Of course, not all the assignments were pleasant, but early on it was apparent the longer-term temp jobs tended to not only be more stable, but actually could open opportunities for permanent employment.

It had been the case on my last long-term situation…at least until several murders proved it an unhealthy place to work.

I'd enjoyed helping, in my own small way, to solve the crimes and see the killer brought to justice. Now my current situation was assisting a mother who needed to deal with her teenage daughter's unexpected health issues while keeping a business operating.

Antique malls have never been places in

which I've spent much time, but I've enjoyed meeting a collection of unique characters who have wares on display in the booths they rent by the month.

The ding of the doorbell ended my musings as I re-entered the mall.

Gerianne gestured me to come over where she stood. "Ms. Newhouse, the Farley sisters wanted to talk with you when you returned. They're at their booth putting in some more items."

"Any idea what they need?"

"Not a clue." Her chirpy voice and attitude boosted my irritation level, which had just been soothed by the latte.

I had no problem with people being cheerful, but some personalities took it to a whole new level.

I tried for a pleasant expression as I veered

left to go to the Farley sisters' booth.

I could only hope they didn't have a complaint I couldn't deal with.

Book available in Soft Cover/Kindle versions on amazon.com

TIME TRAVEL/ END TIMES

SPECIAL EXCERPT

One moment of carelessness – a woman is catapulted into the future to a time and place she never chose. Ruth Blackwell must adapt to life in a millennial society totally foreign to all she's ever known. In her own time, research scientist Derek Ainsley frantically tries to bring her back before the plug is pulled on his time travel experiment. Will he succeed…or be forced to leave her stranded in time forever?

Read on for a portion of Chapter One

Time Out

(Book 1, "Out of Time" series)

by D.A. Featherling

CHAPTER 1

Soaked with perspiration and end-of-day weariness, Ruth Blackwell trudged toward the north parking lot. The campus labyrinth of concrete sidewalks stretched before her, beckoning with the reward of rest and refreshment when she completed the maze.

She swiped at the moisture beading her upper lip. Summer in Texas said it all.

A sudden loud whoop sounded her only warning. Ruth whirled to see two bicycles aimed at her. She braced for the worst.

The riders jinked their fast-moving mountain bikes on the narrow sidewalk.

Crazy kids! They could hit me.

She realized they were aimed at her. On purpose. The bitter, metallic taste of fear watered her mouth. She eyed the distance, sprinted for the stairs.

The first bike raced closer, swerved at the last possible second.

She must keep moving.

The second rider veered, missed her by inches. Her tote bag snagged on the railing, wrenched from her hand onto the sidewalk.

Fountains of nausea surged in her stomach, her vision blurred and dimmed. An adrenaline rush pumped her pulse into double time as she watched the culprits ride on, hooting and flaunting their mastery over their machines.

"Idiots!"

Her yell didn't begin to diffuse her fear or anger. Sucking in a deep breath, she tried to quiet her pounding heart, bent to retrieve her bag. A sudden flood of dizziness washed over her, dropped her to her knees.

A light humming noise resonated in her ears, increased in volume. She must be about to faint.

Nothing happened.

The noise grew louder, concentrated in intensity over her head.

Looking up, Ruth saw a mass of undulating light move downward. Light like nothing she'd ever seen. The waves shimmered faster and faster until they resembled a heat wave rising off July-hot asphalt roads.

She pressed herself against the sidewalk, scrabbled at the unyielding concrete, tried to hide.

Unsuccessful, she raised both hands in a final, feeble attempt to ward off the grasping tentacles of light.

* * * *

Shimon al-Akbar stifled a yawn and scratched one side of his face. His light touch moved over the wrinkles in a near caress as he chewed in slow motion. He watched the younger man who stood across the counter from him.

The man weighed two small stone cups, one in each hand.

Shimon's gaze darted to the clock above the entrance of the small antiquities shop. Almost time to close. Good. Business had crawled again today like it did all week. If the man bought, it would be his only sale of the day. Hopefully tomorrow would prove to be more profitable.

The man placed one of the cups on the counter, held the other out to Shimon. Shimon bowed and took it, pulled a sheet of yellowed paper from under the counter and began to fold the corners over the cup, his wrapping motions automatic.

Glancing past the customer, he looked outside. The glimpse of the street from the dingy shop window showed no signs of life except for one lone figure several buildings away.

To keep their doors open, he and all the other merchants on El Sarir Street needed an influx of rich tourists. Tourists with more money than taste.

During the past several weeks, few of them had strolled through the area or entered the small shops that lined both sides of the narrow street.

Shimon watched for a minute, hoping to see a long line of tourists follow. When none did, he exhaled a mingled scent of onion and spice and returned to his package.

He controlled the urge to spit. Expelling a pungent cardamom seed to emphasize his disgust would be appropriate, but he refrained in deference to the customer standing before him.

He muttered the price, watched while the man fumbled for payment. Shimon's fingers stroked his coarse strands of beard. Tourists always expected him to act the part of the ancient shepherd of the hills.

When he played the role, they assumed his wares were as authentic as his flowing woolen robe, long white whiskers, and wrinkled mahogany skin. People reacted with awe to the persona so only on rare occasions did they bargain with him over his inflated prices.

The customer finally produced a single

coin, handed it to Shimon.

The shopkeeper dropped it into a small box, withdrew two small coins in turn. He inched them across the countertop, avoiding the nicks and cuts in the dull wooden surface.

The man waited, tapped one finger against his package until Shimon finally released the coins.

With a muttered word, indecipherable to the old man, the customer grabbed the money, wheeled and strode out the door into the early evening sun.

Shimon watched him for a moment, heaved a sigh, allowed his gaze to assess his surroundings. A musty odor drifted in the stale air, propelled by the slow-moving blades of the lazy ceiling fan.

Clay pots fraternized with stacks of parchment scrolls. Small hand tools mingled with coins.

So familiar. He could spot a millimeter's movement of any single item. Not that it happened often. He would never get rich from his sales of merchandise, but at his age, he didn't need much to exist. There were few passions left to an old man except survival.

A decrepit brown wooden case with a glass lid contained his most precious goods — odds and ends of metal jewelry from gravesites and tombs.

Small statues of unknown origin littered tables and shelves without discrimination. Stone dishes nestled close to graceful pottery vases.

The dust that overlaid it all contributed its distinct aroma to the character of the murky interior. He couldn't see the powdery residue in the gloom but he knew where it lay. Didn't he spend hours every week dusting, dusting, so his customers wouldn't be offended? A thankless task doomed to failure.

He grinned, felt additional ridges and trenches crease the sides of his face. On the other hand, to some of the tourists, the dust further authenticated his goods.

He peered again at the clock. Another few minutes and he would lock the front door, leave through the back alley and go home to his tiny room a few streets away. Shimon prided himself on staying open daily until the exact time of closing even when the volume of business didn't demand it.

Glancing out the window a second time, the figure seen before now proved to be a slender, brown-haired woman who stood across the street looking at his door. He stiffened. A genuine customer? He squinted.

The woman rubbed her forehead, glanced sideways, then behind her.

Ah, no! She appeared confused or lost. Only someone seeking directions to her companions or her lodging. Not a potential sale. Well, she'd better hurry or his door would be locked. He didn't mind doing a good deed — if convenient.

He shrugged. An arthritic twinge in his shoulder made him wince. He clenched his fist and moved his arm in slow rotation to relieve the pain while he continued to watch.

As though spying his movement, the woman darted across the narrow street toward his shop. The clock hands clicked to the hour of closing as the tinkle of the bell over the door ushered in his visitor.

Book available in Soft Cover/Kindle versions on amazon.com

ROMANTIC COMEDY

SPECIAL EXCERPT

Until she decides to look for a husband, Em Snider is so-o-o-o in control of her life. But her trip on the internet matchmaking highway soon shows her there are toads out there! Em has a chance to discover Prince Charming, if she can survive the shocks. She's soon ready to quit…or will true love still come about in a way she never dreamed if she'll quit stepping on the brakes?

Read on for a portion of Chapter One

Kissing Frogs

(Book 2, "Second Time Around" series)

by D.A. Featherling

CHAPTER 1

It would be a whole lot easier if I could just pick up a tranquilizer gun and bag my quarry with a single shot. Unfortunately, that method is generally frowned upon when husband hunting.

Not that I'm desperate, but after hours and hours on the computer reviewing online dating and matchmaking services, I could get that way fast.

It's all the fault of those ads I saw on TV yesterday. The ones touting an Internet matchmaking service. Very trendy these days.

I watched it with a bit of a sneer curling my upper lip. Romance for a lifetime. Right! This gal has indulged in enough romance – and has the scars to prove it – for this lifetime and probably another one or two as well.

Anyway, nobody wants a fifty-something, independent female for a romantic relationship. At least not anybody I know.

On the other hand….

My reverie is rudely interrupted by a sharp pain in my left ankle.

"Salem, that hurt!" I glare at my unrepentant white Persian whose main mission in life is to remind me who is in charge of this household and call me to order when I don't follow my assigned duties.

His Royalness marches down the hall in arrogant silence toward the kitchen and his meal. I, knowing my place, walk the appropriate humble ten paces behind.

"No wonder I named you Salem." I mutter to make sure he doesn't hear me. "You are such a trial." My ankle twinges in sympathy.

As I automatically open a sack and pour

kitty nuggets, my thoughts return to my Internet search. I turn on the news and sip a cup of coffee.

Not only does this keep Salem from being in my face, but it helps me put my thoughts in order. I change TV channels several times; however, my mind tends to ponder my romance-related thought stream.

After listening to the less-than-inspiring headlines from around the city, state, and world, I turn down the volume. Right now, I couldn't care less about what's happening out there – I have important stuff to decide here.

Alternately thinking and fretting, mid-way through a round of TV channel surfing, I click the remote one more time, and voilà, there's the matchmaking service commercial again. I turn up the sound.

The announcer extols the glorious

adventure of signing up. Scene after scene shows couples billing and cooing, girls with rings on their fingers, and even one older couple under a wedding arch. I wait until the website URL appears, write it down, click off the power. The dilemmas facing the world now seem small in comparison to my own choices.

I'm elated I happened across the ad a second time. I knew I'd seen a lot of those commercials lately. And seen the commercials. And seen the commercials. Ad nauseam. Ad enough.

Perhaps, though, if someone like me finds the right company to use, she'll be in total control of her matrimonial future, not some faceless machine, or worse, a well-meaning friend.

Salem has finished his repast at this point

and wants his personal attention time. No point in fighting it. My ankles will suffer if I don't do as His Highness demands.

I retreat to my recliner and allow my lap to become his pillow, after proper kneading of course.

A tremor of power reverberates in my solar plexus as Salem turns on his motor-like purr.

I scratch the fluffy white fur under his chin, accelerating the rumble.

"Silly cat."

My fingers massage the white head that thrusts, demanding, under my touch.

Cupping Salem's chin in my hand, I glare at his satisfied expression.

"What do you think, boy? Should we get married?"

His baleful look gives me no clues. He jerks away, closes his eyes and goes to sleep.

No help there.

I pull down the footrest on the recliner, dump Salem on the floor. He spits at me. I ignore him and head to the office to spend a bit more time on the computer.

It takes only a few minutes to type in the URL I'd written down earlier. Interesting name – e-marriage.com. Clever without being too cutesy. I click on the link.

Fairly decent looking homepage. I start reading. And clicking. And reading. Twenty minutes later, I sit back and flex my upper body. Hmmm. I'm cautiously optimistic. This might be a possibility. And it doesn't sound like any money is required up front.

They want me to fill out a questionnaire, then they'll send me my profile telling me my strengths and weaknesses. Well, the ones in relationships anyway. They seem to have a pretty safe approach for participants to contact potential whatever-they-call-thems.

I ponder a little more. Click back and forth a couple of pages. Sounds like I can opt out anywhere along the line. If I'm going to be in charge, this sounds like a good way to do it.

Better than becoming one of those frantic, more-than-mature females, who run around dressing like they're twenty, and try to infiltrate underage singles groups at churches to try to convince everybody they're still youthful and marriageable enough for a younger man.

My hand hovers over the mouse. Do it or not? That is the question.

Book available in Soft Cover/Kindle versions on amazon.com

GET UP and GET MOVING!
CHECKLIST

Category	To Do	Begun	Done	Repeat	When Repeat
CLEANING					
House Plants					
Wall Switch Plates					
Frames					
Knick-Knacks					
Shades					
Scatter Rugs					
Mirror Bulbs					
Bathroom					
Mop Floors					
Sweep/Vacuum					

For a FREE 8-1/2 x 11 PDF copy of the checklist of projects, email <u>dafeatherling@gmail.com</u>.

www.ingramcontent.com/pod-product-compliance
Lightning Source LLC
Chambersburg PA
CBHW050033260726

48658CB00005B/1584